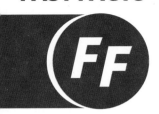

FAST FACTS

Indispensable
Guides to
Clinical
Practice

Colorectal Cancer

Second edition

Irving Taylor
Professor of Surgery and Head of Department,
Chairman of the Academic Division of Surgical
Specialties, Royal Free and University College London
Medical School, University College London, UK

Julio Garcia-Aguilar
Professor of Surgery,
Chief, Section of Colorectal Surgery,
Department of Surgery, University
of California at San Francisco, USA

Stanley M Goldberg
Clinical Professor of Surgery,
Division of Colon and Rectal Surgery, Department of
Surgery, University of Minnesota, Minneapolis, USA

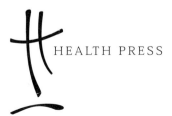

HEALTH PRESS

Oxford

College of the Ouachitas

© Health Press 2000
This local reprint of *Fast Facts - Colorectal Cancer, Second Editon* is
published by arrangement with Health Press Limited

Fast Facts – Colorectal Cancer
First published 1999
Second edition February 2002

Text © Irving Taylor, Julio Garcia-Aguilar, Stanley M Goldberg
© in this edition Health Press Limited
Health Press Limited, Elizabeth House, Queen Street, Abingdon,
Oxford OX14 3JR, UK
Tel: +44 (0)1235 523233
Fax: +44 (0)1235 523238

Fast Facts is a trademark of Health Press Limited.

The publisher and the authors have made every effort to ensure the
accuracy of this book, but cannot accept responsibility for any errors
or omissions.

A CIP catalogue record for this title is available from the British Library.

ISBN 1-903734-08-8

Taylor, I (Irving)
Fast Facts – Colorectal Cancer/
Irving Taylor, Julio Garcia-Aguilar, Stanley M Goldberg

Illustrated by Dee McLean, London, UK.

Typeset by Zed, Oxford, UK.

Printed by Fine Print (Services) Ltd, Oxford, UK.

Introduction

Colorectal cancer remains one of the most common malignancies affecting western civilization. Awareness of the symptoms associated with this disease is extremely important. It can present in a variety of ways, from vague abdominal pain with a change in bowel habit to a major acute emergency with large bowel obstruction, or even with perforation.

In order to achieve the best chance of cure, early diagnosis and appropriate surgical therapy are essential. Unfortunately, diagnosis is often delayed due to vagueness of symptoms and patients' failure to realize the significance of their symptoms. Patients should be referred for investigation and treatment at the earliest opportunity. Surgical treatment is most effective when carried out for localized disease. Once metastases have occurred, the prognosis is significantly worse and palliation may be the only feasible option. Recent developments in chemotherapy and radiotherapy have provided opportunities for adjuvant therapy, and also help in patients with recurrent or advanced disease.

There has been much progress with screening and in the understanding of the genetic changes associated with the development of invasive tumours; this should soon translate into improved therapies. High-risk groups are being identified and may be suitable for regular screening.

The family physician is key in the overall management of patients with colorectal cancer, as well as providing subsequent support services. This new edition of *Fast Facts – Colorectal Cancer* delivers, concisely, the important information required to give an optimal service to patients with this common disorder.

Carcinoma of the large bowel is one of the major malignancies in the western world. In the UK, each year there are 34 000 cases, with a predominance of men over women, and the disease accounts for some 17 000 deaths. In the USA, colorectal cancer is the third most common cancer in both men and women. Incidence in both black and white US men and women gradually increased through most of the 1970s and 1980s. In recent years, incidence rates in black people have overtaken those in white people. Between 1985 and 1993, there were substantial declines in incidence for both white men and white women and the rate for black women may also be starting to decline (Figure 1.1).

Worldwide, the incidence of colorectal cancer varies widely, with a 20-fold variation between different countries for colon cancer and a 10-fold variation for rectal cancer. Incidence of colorectal cancer is apparently lowest in African and Asian countries. There is a well-recognized tendency for migrational convergence to occur, which indicates the importance of recent environmental change. Within the UK, Scotland has a higher rate of

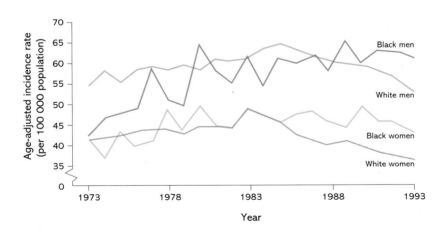

Figure 1.1 Colorectal cancer incidence rates in the USA for black and white men and women.

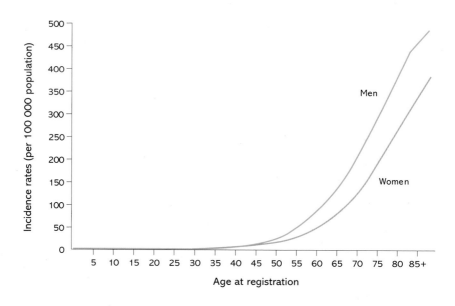

Figure 1.2 Incidence rates by age for colorectal cancer in men and women in the UK.

colon cancer than either England or Wales. The incidence of colorectal cancer increases with age (Figure 1.2).

The distribution of cancers throughout the colon also varies. Tumours on the left side of the colon are common, with sigmoid, rectosigmoid junction and rectal tumours accounting for nearly 70% of cases worldwide (Figure 1.3). The proportion of right-sided colorectal cancers increases with age.

Risk factors

The development of colorectal cancer is thought to be a multifactorial process, involving genetic and environmental factors.

Genetic factors. Recently, a number of mutations within specific genes have been recognized and these are thought to account for the development of colorectal cancer in a high proportion of patients (Figure 1.4).

It is recognized that a mutation in the *Adenomatous Polyposis Coli* (*APC*) gene is responsible for the development of familial adenomatous polyposis (FAP) (see page 31). Thousands of polyps occur throughout the

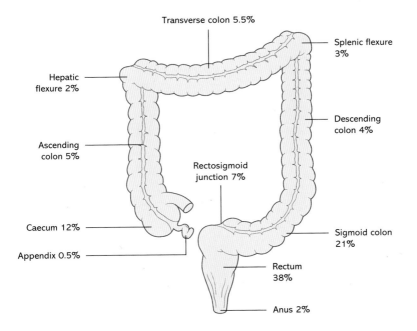

Figure 1.3 Distribution of colorectal cancers throughout the large bowel and rectum. Note the higher incidence on the left side.

colon, with the subsequent development of malignancy. Hereditary non-polyposis colorectal cancer (HNPCC) is also a hereditary syndrome characterized by the familial clustering of colorectal and extracolonic cancers (see page 31). It accounts for 1–3% of all colorectal cancers. Most colorectal cancers are not hereditary, however; they tend to be sporadic and are thought to be due mainly to environmental factors. Nevertheless, certain

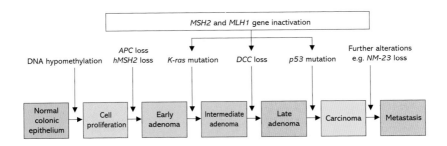

Figure 1.4 Gene mutations responsible for the development of colorectal cancer.

families are at high risk of developing colorectal cancer, and the genetics of these families are being investigated extensively.

Environmental factors. There is much evidence linking the 'western' (high fat content and low fibre intake) diet to the development of colorectal cancer. Interestingly, migrant studies have demonstrated that people who move from low- to high-incidence areas (e.g. Japanese who moved to the USA) also develop the high rates of colorectal cancer associated with their host country. Other environmental factors that may be involved include a high alcohol (particularly beer) intake and obesity.

There is some suggestion that a high calcium intake reduces epithelial proliferation in the gastrointestinal tract, though there is little evidence that calcium in high doses is protective. Other vitamins are thought to have a role in inhibiting malignant transformation by affecting the antioxidants present within the colon.

Although it is difficult to interpret dietary studies, there is evidence that a healthy, well-balanced diet, high in fibre and low in fat and alcohol, may offer some protection. Recently, a number of possible dietary influences have been subjected to investigation (Table 1.1).

Histological features

Colorectal cancer is an adenocarcinoma arising from the epithelial lining of the bowel. Some colorectal cancers may develop *de novo*, but most result from malignant transformation of adenomatous polyps. There are three types of polyps:

TABLE 1.1

Possible dietary factors in colorectal cancer risk

Factor	Examples	Effect
Antioxidants	Vitamins E and C	Protective
Micronutrients	Calcium, folic acid	Protective
Macronutrients	Fat	Promoter
	Fibre	Protective
Food mutagens	Heterocyclic amines	Promoter

- tubular adenomas
- villous adenomas
- tubulovillous adenomas.

Polyps arise from the mucosa and gradually increase in size. Some polyp characteristics – size larger than 1 cm, tubulovillous or villous histology, multiple occurrences – are associated with a high risk of malignant transformation. Most screening programmes are designed to recognize the presence of polyps, or early malignant change in polyps or surrounding mucosa (Figure 1.5).

Staging classifications

There are several different staging classifications for colorectal cancer, but only the Dukes staging from 1932 has stood the test of time:

- Dukes A (confined to the bowel wall)
- Dukes B (involving the full thickness of bowel wall to serosa)
- Dukes C (involvement of mesenteric lymph nodes)
- Dukes D (distant metastatic spread usually to the liver).

The modified Dukes staging and Astler-Coller staging systems are versions of the Dukes classification that take into account spread through the bowel wall and proximal and distal lymph node involvement. More recently, emphasis has been placed on the tumour–nodes–metastases (TNM) classification of colorectal cancer, which gives an indication of the extent of spread (Table 1.2). This classification, though important for colon and rectal cancers of all stages, becomes particularly important in rectal cancer

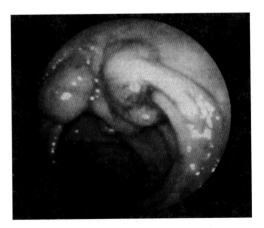

Figure 1.5 Colonoscopic appearance of polyps within the colon showing one polyp on a stalk (pedunculated).

TABLE 1.2

TNM classification of colorectal cancer

Primary tumour (T)
Pathological staging

TX   Primary tumour cannot be assessed

T0   No evidence of primary tumour

Tis Carcinoma *in situ*: intraepithelial
     or invasion of lamina propria*

T1   Tumour invades submucosa

T2   Tumour invades muscularis propria

T3   Tumour invades through the
     muscularis propria into the
     subserosa, or into non-peritonealized
     pericolic or perirectal tissues

T4   Tumour directly invades other
     organs or structures, and/or
     perforates visceral peritoneum†

*Tis includes cancer cells confined within
the glandular basement membrane
(intraepithelial) or lamina propria
(intramucosal) with no extension through
the muscularis mucosa into the submucosa

†Direct invasion in T4 includes invasion of
other segments of the colorectum by way
of the serosa (e.g. invasion of the sigmoid
colon by a carcinoma of the caecum)

Ultrasound staging

uT0 Benign tumour

uT1 Invasion into but not through
     the submucosa

uT2 Invasion into but not through
     the muscularis propria

uT3 Invasion into perirectal fat

uT4 Invasion into adjacent organs

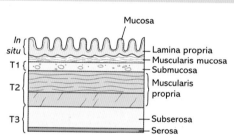

A cross-section through the bowel wall
illustrating the primary tumour (T) section
of the TNM classification.

when local therapies, rather than major ablative surgery, are being
considered (e.g. for a T1 or T2 tumour).

Prognosis. Dukes staging is also important for prognosis. Patients with
Dukes A colorectal cancer have an excellent prognosis whereas those with

Regional lymph nodes (N)

NX Regional lymph nodes cannot be assessed

N0 No regional lymph node metastasis

N1 Metastases in 1 to 3 regional lymph nodes

N2 Metastases in 4 or more regional lymph nodes

uN0 No metastatic perirectal node

uN1 Metastatic perirectal nodes

Distant metastases (M)

MX Distant metastases cannot be assessed

M0 No distant metastasis

M1 Distant metastases

Stage grouping

AJCC/UICC[‡]				Dukes[§]
Stage 0	Tis	N0	M0	–
Stage I	T1	N0	M0	A
	T2	N0	M0	–
Stage II	T3	N0	M0	B
	T4	N0	M0	–
Stage III	Any T	N1	M0	C
	Any T	N2	M0	–
Stage IV	Any T	Any N	M1	D

[‡]American Joint Committee on Cancer/International Union Against Cancer

[§]Dukes B is a composite of better (T3/N0/M0) and worse (T4/N0/M0) prognostic groups, as is Dukes C (Any T/N1/M0 and Any T/N2/M0)

Dukes C have a much worse prognosis (Figure 1.6). Unfortunately, the incidence of Dukes A colorectal cancer is less than 10% compared with 45% for Dukes C colorectal cancer. Approximately 25% of patients present with Dukes D colorectal cancer, and few of these patients survive for 3 years.

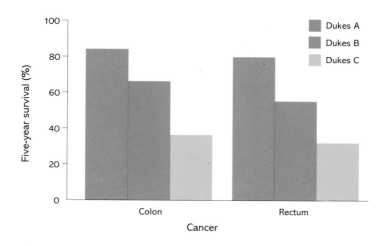

Figure 1.6 Prognosis for colorectal cancer related to Dukes staging.

The differentiation (the degree of similarity of tumour architecture to the structure of the organ from which the tumour arose) of colorectal cancer also has an important role in determining prognosis. Tumours are divided into:

• well differentiated
• moderately differentiated
• poorly differentiated
• anaplastic.

Overall prognosis can be correlated to the degree of differentiation. A well-differentiated tumour will have a relatively good prognosis whereas the anaplastic state is typical of a rapidly growing malignant tumour.

Pattern of spread

Large bowel cancer is locally invasive. It spreads through the full thickness of the bowel wall into adjacent tissues. Symptoms of obstruction occur as the lumen of the bowel is occluded (Chapter 6). However, metastatic spread may be evident before local growth produces symptoms.

The most common site of metastases is the liver. Approximately 25% of patients have liver metastases present at the time of colorectal resection, and approximately 50% of all other patients will subsequently develop liver metastases (Chapter 7). Other sites of metastatic spread are the lungs, brain and bones, but these are unusual in the absence of liver metastases. Patients may also develop peritoneal spread with the formation of malignant ascites.

Prognosis is significantly better when colorectal cancer is diagnosed and treated at an early stage. The disease tends to progress in a logical fashion from benign to malignant lesions, and then to metastatic spread. It is far better to treat a patient early, with the expectation of cure, than to cope with the serious effects of metastatic involvement.

A detailed history and examination will often reveal the site of malignancy within the large bowel or rectum. Patients with colorectal cancer can develop a myriad of symptoms as highlighted below.

Abdominal pain

Frequently, abdominal pain is non-specific and may be localized to any quadrant of the abdomen or be diffuse. When the pain is persistent and colicky, it is more likely to represent obstructive symptoms and be due to a lesion in the descending colon. More localized tenderness with signs of localized peritonitis indicates local invasion of the adjacent peritoneum. It is uncommon for colorectal cancer to perforate the bowel, but when it does the prognosis is significantly worse. Patients with persistent perineal pain associated with tenesmus are more likely to have a large rectal cancer. It can be difficult to distinguish the pain associated with diverticular disease from that due to a carcinoma in the sigmoid or descending colon. Patients with diverticular disease can also have an underlying carcinoma, and investigation of this patient group is therefore very important.

Change in bowel habit

Any patient over the age of 45 with an alteration in bowel habit that lasts for more than 2 weeks should probably be investigated. The change in bowel habit might be diarrhoea, which may be bloody, possibly associated with a sense of incomplete defecation. Patients frequently complain of diarrhoea when they are actually suffering from incomplete defecation, a symptom often associated with tenesmus. These latter symptoms indicate a rectal tumour. Patients with constipation and associated colicky abdominal pain may have an underlying obstructive lesion and should be investigated.

Alternating diarrhoea and constipation associated with colicky abdominal pain is uncommon; this indicates a subacute, large bowel obstruction.

Rectal bleeding

Rectal bleeding is common and often associated with haemorrhoids. Bleeding from haemorrhoids is usually bright red with accompanying anal discomfort. The bleeding is intermittent and splashes the toilet pan.

Rectal bleeding that is darker in colour and mixed in with stool is more indicative of bleeding secondary to an underlying carcinoma. Rectal bleeding associated with tenesmus should be investigated urgently. Patients with a recent development of rectal bleeding should be examined carefully, particularly if over 45 years of age, to exclude the presence of an underlying rectal cancer. Rectal bleeding always demands diagnostic investigation.

Anaemia

The development of non-specific anaemia of 'unknown origin' is not uncommon in patients with a carcinoma in the ascending colon. As these patients rarely have abdominal pain, they present with advanced disease. Bleeding is occult and may be recognized on faecal occult blood testing of the stools. Anaemia is iron deficient and microcytic. In the UK, often the initial investigation of such patients is by gastroscopy as an upper gastrointestinal disorder is suspected. If this proves normal, the next most logical investigation is colonoscopy. In the USA, however, patients with non-specific anaemia tend to be initially examined with colonoscopy as carcinoma of the right colon is believed to be 'silent'.

Anorexia and weight loss

Anorexia and weight loss frequently accompany colorectal cancer and are often associated with advanced disease. The differential diagnosis in these patients is a gastric carcinoma, but when investigations are negative it is important to exclude a large bowel malignancy.

Early diagnosis

The earlier diagnosis is made and treatment initiated, the better the prognosis. In the UK, guidelines have been introduced to highlight specific symptoms that indicate more rapid referral to a specialist team. Symptoms include:
- rectal bleeding with a change in bowel habit
- rectal bleeding without anal symptoms

- change in bowel habit, including increased frequency and loose stools for several weeks
- those that indicate intestinal obstruction (colicky abdominal pain, distension, constipation).

Examination

Features on clinical examination that provide a suspicion of malignancy include:

- anaemia (haemoglobin < 10 g/dl)
- abdominal masses.

A mass in the right iliac fossa indicates extensive caecal or ascending colon carcinoma (Figure 2.1), whereas a mass in the left iliac fossa indicates sigmoid carcinoma. Rectal examination can reveal a carcinoma of the rectum, and masses may be palpated in the Pouch of Douglas or anteriorly in males. This indicates either a carcinoma within the sigmoid colon or peritoneal metastases within the pelvis.

On rectal examination, the degree of fixity of a tumour is important and may have a bearing on subsequent treatment. It is occasionally difficult to

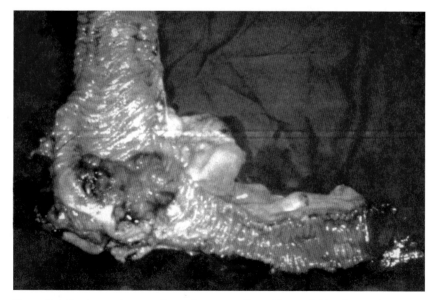

Figure 2.1 Carcinoma in ascending colon presenting with occult bleeding and anaemia.

TABLE 2.1

Symptoms of colorectal cancer

Right colon	Left colon
• Little pain	• Often colicky pain
• Weight loss	• Weight loss less common
• Occult bleeding	• Rectal bleeding
• Obstructive symptoms uncommon	• Obstructive symptoms and signs
• Mass in right iliac fossa	• Mass in left iliac fossa
• Change in bowel habit uncommon	• Change in bowel habit is an early symptom
• Higher proportion of Dukes C	• Less advanced disease on presentation

distinguish a rectal cancer from a prostate or fixed cervical malignancy, but biopsy should assist in this regard.

It is often possible to distinguish cancers on the right side of the colon from cancers on the left side by means of symptomatology and clinical examination (Table 2.1).

Jaundice and hepatomegaly indicate advanced disease with extensive liver metastases and are harbingers of a very poor prognosis. Often they occur in the presence of ascites, indicating peritoneal metastases.

Rarer clinical signs of an underlying colorectal cancer include:
• pneumaturia
• gastro-colic fistula
• ischiorectal or perineal abscesses which indicate underlying rectal cancer
• deep venous thrombosis.

Differential diagnosis. Careful history and examination can exclude:
• diverticular disease
• irritable bowel syndrome
• inflammatory bowel disease

- local rectal pathology (e.g. haemorrhoids)
- ischaemic colitis
- pneumatosis coli.

Nevertheless, further investigation is frequently necessary to provide definitive evidence of an underlying carcinoma.

Confirmation of the diagnosis requires examination of the entire colon. Colorectal cancer staging is based on the use of imaging studies and pathological examination of the resected specimen. Accurate staging is essential for the selection of patients who may benefit from adjuvant therapy and for determining prognosis.

Diagnosis of the primary tumour

Any patient with a clinical history suggesting colorectal cancer should undergo examination of the entire colon. The goal is to diagnose the primary lesion and to exclude any synchronous polyps or cancers. Traditionally, this has been accomplished by colonoscopy or barium enema. More recently, enhanced-resolution spiral computed tomography (CT) has enabled CT colography (CT pneumocolon) to be performed with a high degree of sensitivity and specificity (Figure 3.1).

Colonoscopy provides high-resolution images of the lesion (Figure 3.2) and allows the performance of diagnostic (biopsy) or therapeutic (polypectomy) interventions. However, colonoscopy is uncomfortable for the patient and requires conscious sedation. It is technically demanding and in 10% of patients, it cannot be completed to the caecum. Respiratory

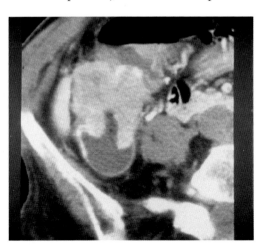

Figure 3.1 CT pneumocolon demonstrating obstructing carcinoma of ascending colon.

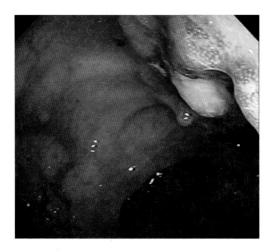

Figure 3.2 Colonoscopy showing carcinoma in rectum.

depression is not uncommon, and colonic perforation occurs in 0.17% of the patients. Rigid sigmoidoscopy is able to visualize the rectum and rectosigmoid region, but not the more proximal colon.

Double-contrast barium enema is cheaper and safer than colonoscopy, and can image the entire colon in almost 100% of cases. Barium enema is less sensitive than colonoscopy in detecting polyps smaller than 5 mm diameter, but the sensitivity of both techniques is similar (95%) for lesions greater than 1 cm diameter. With barium enema, it is not possible to take a biopsy of the tumour or snare polyps (Figure 3.3).

In general, colonoscopy should be the diagnostic test of choice in most patients suspected of having colorectal cancer. Double-contrast barium

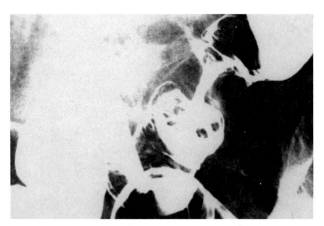

Figure 3.3 Barium enema showing typical carcinoma ('apple-core' stricture) in descending colon.

enema should be performed when colonoscopy is not successful in reaching the caecum. This can often be done on the same day, to spare the patient a new bowel preparation.

Diagnosis of metastatic disease

The optimal surgical treatment of colon cancer demands resection of the segment of the colon containing the tumour and the lymph nodes draining that segment of the bowel. In general, the extent of resection in colon cancer is independent of the stage of the tumour. To avoid devastating complications such as large bowel obstruction, haemorrhage or tumour perforation, the primary tumour is usually resected even in the presence of distant metastases. However, in patients with a short life expectancy due to poor general condition or extensive metastatic disease, a non-surgical approach or a less radical resection may be indicated.

Therefore, there is not a consensus on the degree of pre-operative evaluation that is necessary to exclude metastatic disease. A standard pre-operative chest radiograph is useful for the detection of pulmonary metastases. Liver ultrasound or CT should be performed. An abdominal CT scan may demonstrate tumour involvement of adjacent organs, suggesting the need for a more radical resection, or it may identify extensive metastatic involvement of the liver, assisting the surgeon to decide on the most effective procedure. Recently, positron emission tomography (PET) has been shown to be very effective in the recognition of small metastatic deposits, particularly in the liver (Figure 3.4).

Pre-operative staging of rectal cancer

In properly selected patients, transanal excision of early rectal cancer results in tumour control equivalent to that obtained with radical surgery, but without the need for major abdominal operation or a permanent colostomy. However, only anatomically accessible tumours that are localized to the bowel wall are candidates for local excision with curative intent. Once the tumour has spread into the perirectal fat or the regional lymph nodes, it cannot be cured by local excision alone. Therefore, pre-operative determination of the depth of mural invasion and the nodal status is critical in patient selection for local excision. The depth of mural invasion is particularly important because it is directly related to the incidence of

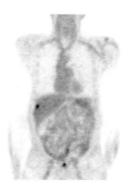

Figure 3.4 Coronal PET image of liver showing solitary 'hotspot' representing liver metastasis from colorectal primary.

lymph node involvement, local recurrence and 5-year survival. Local and regional staging of rectal cancer relies primarily on four techniques:
- digital rectal examination
- endorectal ultrasound
- CT scanning
- magnetic resonance imaging (MRI).

Digital rectal examination is only useful for tumours located in the distal portion of the rectum and permits only a gross estimation of depth of invasion. Accuracy of staging by digital examination varies significantly with the experience of the examiner. When correlated with pathological staging, digital examination identifies extrarectal invasion with reasonable accuracy, but fails to discriminate the degree of intramural invasion. Digital examination also fails to identify more than 50% of the pathologically proven involved nodes. Therefore, digital rectal examination is more accurate in staging locally-advanced rather than early tumours, and thus its value in selecting patients for local therapy is limited.

Endorectal ultrasound provides a 360° cross-sectional image of the rectum and perirectal tissue, and is able to discriminate the different layers of the rectal wall (Figure 3.5). The accuracy of endorectal ultrasound for determining the depth of rectal wall invasion ranges from 81 to 94%. The accuracy for detecting lymph node metastases ranges from 58 to 86%. A modification of the TNM staging, with degrees of invasion that

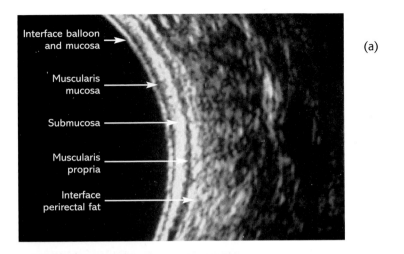

(a)

Interface balloon and mucosa →

Muscularis mucosa

Submucosa

Muscularis propria

Interface perirectal fat

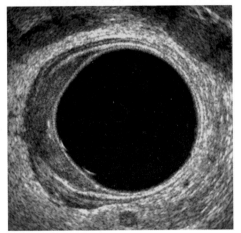

(b)

Figure 3.5 Endorectal ultrasound scans: (a) detail of the different layers of the rectal wall, (b) tumour penetrating into the perirectal fat with a metastatic perirectal lymph node.

correspond very closely to the pathological stages, is currently used for the pre-operative ultrasonographic staging of rectal tumours (see Table 1.2, pages 12 and 13). Ultrasonographic classification (uT0–uT4) is used in decision-making.

CT scanning and MRI show extrarectal invasion and invasion of contiguous organs better than endorectal ultrasonography, but they cannot distinguish the individual layers of the bowel wall (Figure 3.6). They are less useful than endorectal ultrasound in the selection of patients for local therapy. A CT scan is less accurate than endorectal ultrasound in the

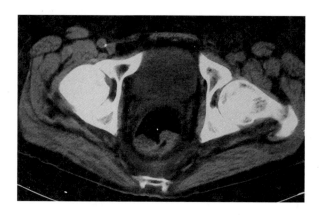

Figure 3.6 CT scan of rectum showing extensive invasion of tumours into adjacent soft tissues.

diagnosis of lymph node metastasis. Abdominal CT is useful in detecting retroperitoneal lymph nodes and liver metastasis. It is used primarily in the selection of patients with advanced tumours for adjuvant pre-operative treatment.

Most colorectal cancers develop from benign adenomatous polyps. The transformation of normal colonic mucosa to an invasive carcinoma is the result of the accumulation of mutations in oncogenes and tumour suppressor genes over several years (Chapter 1). The slow development of a colorectal cancer provides a window of opportunity for the detection and removal of premalignant adenomatous polyps and early-stage cancers. Evidence accumulated in the past few years demonstrates that the removal of adenomatous polyps reduces the incidence of cancer, and that diagnosis of colorectal cancers at earlier stages decreases mortality.

Screening methods

These include:

- faecal occult blood (FOB) tests
- sigmoidoscopy
- combined FOB test and flexible sigmoidoscopy
- colonoscopy
- barium enema.

Faecal occult blood test. Colorectal cancers and polyps bleed more than the normal mucosa. Bleeding is usually intermittent, but the chance of bleeding is proportional to the size of the tumour. Detection of tumour bleeding is the basis of the most widely used screening test: the guaiac-based detection of the pseudoperoxidase activity of haemoglobin in the stool. The FOB test involves smearing two samples of stool on to the window of a card that contains the guaiac reagent (Figure 4.1). Some foods can cause a false-positive reaction, so a special diet must be followed for 2 days prior to the test.

The test is repeated on three consecutive stool samples. It is not specific for cancer; bleeding from any other source will give a positive result. As most tumours bleed slowly and intermittently, the sensitivity of the test is low. Methods aimed at increasing the sensitivity, such as rehydrating the cards, reduce the specificity of the test. The sensitivity of the test increases

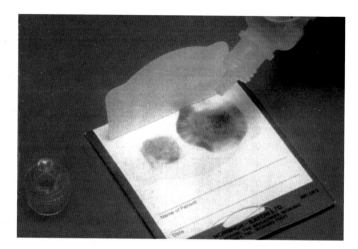

Figure 4.1
Test for faecal
occult blood.

with the number of samples tested, and therefore testing of stool samples
from several consecutive days is recommended. A positive FOB test
(Figure 4.2) should be followed by total colonic evaluation with
colonoscopy. Several prospective randomized trials have demonstrated that
screening by FOB testing reduces the mortality from colorectal cancer.

Sigmoidoscopy. Flexible sigmoidoscopy with a 60 cm scope can detect
40–60% of all colorectal cancers and polyps. The procedure is fast,
requires minimal preparation, and is relatively well tolerated by patients.
The presence of adenomatous polyps in the rectosigmoid colon increases the

Figure 4.2
Guaiac-based
test showing
positive result
for faecal
occult blood.

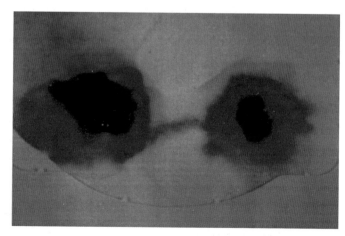

probability of finding additional polyps or cancers in more proximal segments of the large bowel. Therefore, if an adenomatous polyp is found during a flexible sigmoidoscopy, the patient should undergo a complete colonoscopy. Several case-control studies have demonstrated that screening by sigmoidoscopy reduces mortality from colorectal cancer. There is evidence for down-staging of cancers found at screening compared with controls, and a 15–20% improvement in 5-year survival when screening is carried out biannually. For instance, in the Nottingham study 51% of the screened group had Dukes A carcinoma compared with 11% in the control group.

Combined faecal occult blood test and flexible sigmoidoscopy. Although the evidence for combining the FOB test and flexible sigmoidoscopy is weaker than for each test separately, it has the theoretical advantage of detecting lesions located throughout the colon. Annual FOB testing combined with flexible sigmoidoscopy every 5 years is becoming the screening method of choice for the average-risk population.

Colonoscopy is the most effective procedure for the diagnosis of colorectal polyps and cancers, but its efficacy as a screening test for colorectal cancer has not been tested in a prospective randomized trial. However, there is good indirect evidence indicating that a full colonoscopy performed at 10-year intervals will reduce the mortality from colorectal cancer.

Barium enema. Double-contrast barium enema can detect most of the clinically important lesions in the colon, but, as with colonoscopy, its effectiveness as a screening test for colorectal cancer is based only on indirect evidence. A double-contrast barium enema every 5–10 years should provide the same degree of protection as the other screening strategies.

Detection of altered DNA in the stool. Colorectal cancer screening by detection of altered DNA from exfoliated tumour cells is currently under investigation.

Risk factors

Three-quarters of colorectal cancers occur in people who do not have any special predisposing factors and therefore are considered at average risk for

29

College of the Ouachitas

TABLE 4.1

Risk factors for colorectal cancer

- Family history of colorectal neoplasia
  - carcinoma
  - adenoma (< 60 years of age)
- Past history of colorectal neoplasm
  - carcinoma
  - adenoma
- Inflammatory bowel disease
  - chronic ulcerative colitis
  - Crohn's disease

- Familial adenomatous polyposis
  - Gardner's syndrome
  - Turcot's syndrome
  - attenuated polyposis
- Hereditary non-polyposis colorectal cancer
- Juvenile polyposis
- Hamartomas

colorectal cancer. The remaining 25% of patients have risk factors that predispose them to the development of colorectal cancer (Table 4.1).

Family history. First-degree relatives of patients with colorectal cancer or polyps have an increased risk of developing colorectal cancer. The severity of the risk increases with the number of relatives affected and with an early age of cancer diagnosis.

Previous history of colorectal cancer. Compared with people with average risk, patients surviving a colorectal cancer have four times the lifetime risk of developing a new (metachronous) colorectal cancer.

Inflammatory bowel disease. Patients with ulcerative colitis and Crohn's disease are at higher risk for the development of colorectal cancer than the general population. The risk is highest among patients diagnosed with inflammatory bowel disease at an early age, with disease extending proximal to the splenic flexure, and with disease lasting longer than 8 years. The colorectal cancers associated with inflammatory disease often do not develop from benign adenomatous polyps, but from flat areas of dysplasia. This makes early diagnosis particularly difficult. However, less than 1% of all colorectal cancers are associated with inflammatory bowel disease.

Hamartomas. Patients with hereditary syndromes characterized by the presence of hamartomas in the small and large bowel are at increased risk for the development of colorectal cancer. However, the magnitude of the increase is unknown.

Hereditary colorectal cancer syndromes. Familial adenomatous polyposis is an autosomal dominant disease characterized by the development of hundreds or thousands of adenomatous polyps throughout the large bowel in the teens or early twenties (see Chapter 1). If untreated, FAP patients will develop colorectal cancer in the fourth or fifth decade of life. This disease is responsible for 1% of all colorectal cancers. The disease has several phenotypic variants such as Gardner's syndrome (familial colorectal cancer, osteomas and desmoid tumours), Turcot's syndrome (familial colorectal cancer and brain tumours), and attenuated familial adenomatous polyposis (less than 100 polyps developing later in life). The FAP syndrome is the result of a mutation of the APC gene. The variable location of the mutation within the gene is responsible for the different phenotypic variants of the disease.

The HNPCC syndrome is characterized by the development of colorectal cancers at an early age. The syndrome is caused by a mutation in the genes coding for proteins responsible for correction of errors in DNA replication. The syndrome often features multiple synchronous cancers, which are frequently located proximal to the splenic flexure. Some patients have an increased incidence of extracolonic malignancies (upper gastrointestinal, urological and female reproductive tract). In contrast to the polyposis that is pathognomonic for FAP, there is no phenotypic marker for HNPCC. Therefore, the diagnosis of HNPCC is based on family history. The diagnostic criteria for HNPCC, known as the Amsterdam criteria, include:

- the existence of three or more relatives with colorectal cancer, one of whom is a first-degree relative of the other two
- the involvement of at least two consecutive generations
- at least one patient being younger than 50 years of age.

The Amsterdam Criteria II include the extracolonic tumours commonly observed in HNPCC, such as cancer of the endometrium, urinary tract and upper gastrointestinal tract.

TABLE 4.2

Colorectal cancer screening and surveillance recommendations

	Risk category	Recommendation
Average risk • 65–75% of CRC • Lifetime risk 5%	• Everyone aged 50 and above without other risk factors	• FOB test plus flexible sigmoidoscopy **or** • Total examination of the colon (if requested and the implications understood) *
Moderate risk • 20–30% of CRC • Lifetime risk 10–30%	• One first-degree relative with CRC or polyps diagnosed > 60	• Average-risk screen • Colonoscopy
	• One first-degree relative with CRC or polyps diagnosed < 60 **or** • Two first-degree relatives any age	• Colonoscopy
	• Prior neoplastic polyp (> 1 cm, proximal or multiple)	• Colonoscopy
	• Single diminutive polyp (< 1 cm)	• Colonoscopy
	• History of curative-intent resection for CRC	• Colonoscopy
	• Inflammatory bowel disease	• Colonoscopy with surveillance biopsies for dysplasia
High risk • 5–8% of CRC • Lifetime risk 50%	• Familial adenomatous polyposis: child or sibling of affected patient	• Sigmoidoscopy • Referral to specialists • Genetic testing
	• Hereditary non-polyposis colorectal cancer: at-risk patient whose family fits Amsterdam criteria or positive gene test	• Colonoscopy • Offer genetic testing • Gynaecological screening for women

*The UK and USA differ

Age to begin (years)	Interval
• 50	• Annual FOB test
	• Flexible sigmoidoscopy every 5 years
	• Colonoscopy every 10 years
	or
	• Double-contrast barium enema + flexible sigmoidoscopy every 5–10 years
• Average-risk screen: 40	• Same as above until first colonoscopy
• Colonoscopy: 50	• Follow-up colonoscopies every 5 years
• 40	• Every 5 years for negative examination
or	
• 10 years before youngest case in the family	
• 3 years after initial polypectomy	• 3 years if more polyps found
	• 5-year interval for normal examination
• 5 years after polypectomy	• 3 years if more polyps found
	• 5-year interval for normal examination
• At time of resection, a total colon examination should be done	• 1 and 3 years after resection
	then
	• 5 years for normal examination
• 8 years after start of pancolitis	• Every 1–2 years
• 12–15 years after left-sided colitis	• Colectomy is recommended for any dysplasia
• 12 if patient is at risk or carrier	• Annually until colectomy (performed if polyps appear)
• Upper GI endoscopy every 1–2 years after diagnosis	
• 21	• Every 2 years until age 40
	then
	• Annually

Screening recommendations

Patients with symptoms of colorectal cancer are not candidates for screening and should undergo the appropriate diagnostic studies. In the general population, screening recommendations are based on individual risk assessment (Table 4.2).

Average risk. If requested and the implications understood, people at average risk for the development of colorectal cancer (asymptomatic males and females above the age of 50 years without risk factors) could undergo yearly FOB testing combined with flexible sigmoidoscopy every 5 years. Patients with a positive FOB test or a polyp identified by flexible sigmoidoscopy should have the entire colon and rectum examined by colonoscopy. Double-contrast barium enema every 5–10 years or colonoscopy every 10 years are accepted screening alternatives in the average-risk population. A digital rectal examination should be performed at the time of sigmoidoscopy or colonoscopy in all individuals.

Moderate risk. Screening should start at age 40, or 10 years before the youngest case in the family, whichever is earlier, in individuals:
- with a first-degree relative with colorectal cancer or polyps before the age of 60

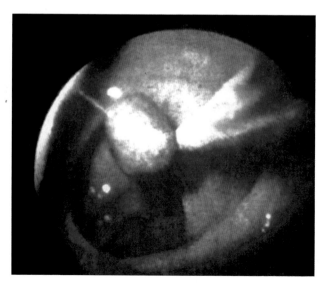

Figure 4.3 Local polypectomy for polyp in sigmoid colon indicated by positive faecal occult blood test.

- with more than one first-degree relative with colorectal cancer or polyps at any age.

Colonoscopy should be repeated every 5 years.

Patients undergoing endoscopic excision of a small (< 1 cm) adenomatous polyp (Figure 4.3) should have the entire colon examined at the time of the polypectomy and have the colonoscopy repeated in 5 years. If the test is negative, they should follow average-risk screening recommendations.

Patients with a large (> 1 cm) adenomatous polyp who have their entire colon examined at the time of the polypectomy should have their colon examined 3 years later and, if normal, every 5 years thereafter.

A complete colonic examination should be carried out pre-operatively in patients undergoing curative resection for colorectal cancer. The colonoscopy should be repeated at 1 and 3 years after surgery, and every 5 years thereafter if the previous one was normal.

Patients with inflammatory bowel disease should undergo colonoscopy with surveillance biopsies for dysplasia 8 years after pancolitis starts, or 12–15 years after the diagnosis of left-sided colitis. Colonoscopy should be repeated every 1–2 years. Patients with dysplasia should undergo colectomy.

High risk. This category includes individuals from families diagnosed as having hereditary forms of colorectal cancer.

A sibling or a child of an FAP patient should start surveillance by flexible sigmoidoscopy at puberty. After the diagnosis is established, the patient should undergo colectomy or a yearly colonoscopy until colectomy. Upper gastrointestinal endoscopy should be performed every 1–2 years.

Individuals from families fitting the Amsterdam criteria for HNPCC should have a colonoscopy at 21 years of age. Follow-up colonoscopy should be performed every 2 years until the age of 40, and yearly thereafter. Genetic counselling and testing should be considered in both circumstances.

At-risk members of families having hereditary cancer syndromes should be informed about the benefits and limitations of genetic counselling and genetic testing.

Consequences of screening

The full spectrum of clinical consequences of screening, other than the prevention of colorectal cancer deaths, is difficult to predict because every screening strategy initiates a cascade of events, each one with uncertain probability. The rate of false-positive tests, the number of colonoscopies performed, the complication of the screening and diagnostic tests, and the number of patients that may require surveillance as a consequence of screening are complex events that happen at different times over several decades. However, cost-effectiveness analysis in the USA has demonstrated that screening for colorectal cancer in average-risk patients is within the range of the cost-effectiveness of other screening tests. However, the situation in the UK and USA differs somewhat. In the UK, there is less emphasis on screening for colorectal cancer, and few people with average risk undergo routine screening. Pilot studies have been undertaken in selected districts to assess the overall cost–benefit analysis of FOB and flexible sigmoidoscopic population screening.

Implementation of guidelines

Awareness of the risks of colorectal cancer and its symptoms is low in the general population, and therefore the number of individuals participating in screening programmes is low. The spread of information among patients is an essential part of the screening programme. Primary-care physicians have the responsibility to inform their patients about their risk of colorectal cancer, the benefits of screening and the different strategies, and to set up a system to implement these guidelines.

Treatment of colorectal cancer is primarily surgical. Anatomical considerations affect the surgical technique and adjuvant therapy, so the treatment of cancers located above or below the peritoneal reflection should be considered separately. Some aspects, however, such as diagnostic evaluation and pre-operative preparation, apply equally to cancers in both colon and rectum.

Pre-operative preparation

The patient should undergo adequate pre-operative evaluation to:
- confirm the diagnosis
- exclude synchronous colorectal cancer or polyps
- determine the local and regional extent of the disease
- exclude the presence of distant metastases
- investigate their overall medical condition, paying particular attention to continence.

The colon harbours the largest numbers of bacteria, mostly anaerobes, in the gastrointestinal tract. Sepsis, both incisional and intra-abdominal, secondary to spillage of faecal matter, is a potential complication of colorectal surgery. Therefore, the reduction of the bacterial load in the colon is one of the most important aspects of the pre-operative management. Current methods combine mechanical preparation and antibiotics.

Colon cancer

Surgery. At the time of performing the laparotomy, it is important to examine the entire peritoneal cavity to exclude metastatic disease, particularly in the liver, omentum and pelvis. The small bowel is also inspected for any unsuspected pathology. Curative surgical treatment of colon cancer requires resection of the segment of the intestine harbouring the tumour, the adjacent mesentery containing the draining lymph nodes, and any organ or tissue adherent to the tumour. Most adhesions between the tumour and adjacent organs are inflammatory, but tumour infiltration cannot be excluded before resection. Infiltration to adjacent organs reduces the chances of cure.

The lymphatics draining the bowel run parallel to the mesenteric blood vessels. The extent of surgical resection depends on the location of the tumour in relation to the major blood vessels (Figure 5.1). When the colon has been adequately prepared, intestinal continuity can be re-established by either a hand-sewn or stapled anastomosis. If more than one cancer is present in different segments of the colon, or when the cancer is associated with multiple neoplastic polyps, a subtotal colectomy with ileorectal anastomosis may be considered.

Patients found to have metastatic disease at the time of surgery should undergo a palliative resection to prevent obstruction and haemorrhage from the primary tumour. In this situation, an extensive mesenteric resection is not usually necessary. Occasionally, a bypass procedure is the only possibility.

After the operation, the bowel is maintained at rest until the ileus resolves. A nasogastric tube is not routinely used in the postoperative period. The most common postoperative complications are:

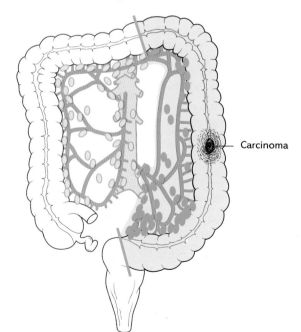

Figure 5.1 Extent of resection of carcinoma of the descending or sigmoid colon.

Carcinoma

- atelectasis
- urinary tract infection
- deep venous thrombosis
- incisional wound infection
- anastomotic dehiscence.

Adjuvant therapy. Survival after curative resection for colon cancer is directly related to the pathological stage of the disease. Patients with tumours localized to the bowel wall (stage I) have a relatively good prognosis, with a 5-year survival greater than 80%. Adjuvant systemic chemotherapy is not recommended for patients with stage I disease.

Stage II or Dukes B disease. Several studies conducted in the USA and Europe have demonstrated no survival advantages for patients with stage II colon cancer treated by surgery plus chemotherapy, compared with surgery alone. Consequently, postoperative chemotherapy is not routinely recommended for patients with stage II colon cancer. However, patients with stage II cancers that are perforated, have close margins, or have undifferentiated histology, may be individually considered for adjuvant chemotherapy, and if possible entered into a trial.

Stage III or Dukes C disease. In patients with lymph node metastases undergoing resection alone, the 5-year survival drops to 25–75%, depending on the differentiation of the tumour, degree of bowel wall invasion, and number of involved lymph nodes. Results from various prospective studies indicate that stage III colon cancer patients benefit from postoperative adjuvant chemotherapy. The agents most commonly used are fluorouracil and leucovorin (folinic acid). Six monthly cycles of chemotherapy given on the first week of each cycle improves survival by 33%. The addition of other drugs effective in advanced disease, such as irinotecan and oxaliplatin, is currently under investigation in prospective trials.

Monoclonal antibodies are undergoing assessment in clinical trials. 17-1A (Panorex) proved interesting in early studies, but more-recent randomized trials have failed to demonstrate major survival benefit.

Portal vein cytotoxic infusion. In patients with resected colon cancer, portal vein infusion with fluorouracil is undergoing assessment. There is evidence to suggest that curatively resected colon (but not rectal) cancer is associated with a survival improvement.

Future adjuvant chemotherapy regimens. There is increasing evidence to suggest that molecular and genetic features of the primary tumour, including the presence of microsatellite instability and retention of heterozygosity, could predict which patients are likely to respond favourably to adjuvant systemic chemotherapy. It is likely that future studies will include such criteria in their protocols.

Rectal cancer

Most rectal cancers are adenocarcinomas biologically indistinguishable from colon cancers; they originate from premalignant lesions, penetrate the bowel wall and the lymphatics in the same fashion, and metastasize to the same organs. Treatment is also primarily surgical. However, some anatomical features give the physician more diagnostic possibilities and alternative therapies for the management of patients with rectal cancer, including:

- extraperitoneal location within the confines of the pelvis
- anatomical relationship to the urogenital system
- dual blood supply from the mesenteric and iliac vessels
- proximity to the anal sphincter mechanism
- complex physiological function
- accessibility.

Surgical treatment of rectal cancer requires consideration of tumour characteristics, such as size, location, depth of invasion, nodal status, differentiation, and patient-related factors, such as co-morbid conditions, anorectal functional status and patient desires. Pre-operative evaluation should include a:

- complete medical history and physical evaluation
- digital examination to determine the functional status of the anal sphincter and the fixity of distal tumours
- proctoscopic exam to assess the size and location of the tumours
- colonoscopy to diagnose any synchronous neoplastic lesion.

An abdominal and pelvic CT can determine the extent of perirectal involvement and the presence of liver metastasis. If available, an endorectal ultrasound is useful to define the tumour penetration of the bowel wall and the presence of perirectal lymph node metastasis.

Radical surgery. At diagnosis, most rectal cancers have already spread beyond the rectal wall, either by direct extension or lymphatic spread, and require radical resection. The radical surgical treatment of rectal cancer should follow the classic oncological principles of removing the site of the primary tumour and the regional lymph nodes.

The rectum should be removed en bloc with the surrounding mesenteric fat harbouring the blood vessels and lymphatics, known as the mesorectum. The superior rectal artery should be ligated distal to the take-off of the left colic artery. Involvement of the lateral or circumferential resection margin is strongly correlated with the later development of local recurrence. Therefore, most surgeons now advocate complete excision of the mesorectum. The hypogastric nerves should be identified and preserved. A margin of at least 1–2 cm of normal rectum distal to the tumour should be included to reduce the risk of anastomotic recurrence. As with colon cancer, any adhesion to adjacent organs, such as the uterus, vagina, bladder or small bowel, should be resected en bloc with the rectum. Restoration of intestinal continuity is an important but secondary consideration. It should only be attempted if a well-perfused, tension-free anastomosis can be performed (low anterior resection, Figure 5.2). When the cancer is so low that the 2 cm margin cannot be obtained without compromising the sphincter function, the entire rectum and anus should be removed (abdominoperineal resection) and a permanent colostomy created (Figure 5.3).

Localized disease. A growing number of patients are diagnosed while their cancer is still localized in the rectal wall (stage I or Dukes A). Studies have demonstrated that, in properly selected patients (Figure 5.4), several forms of local therapy (transanal local excision, endocavitary radiation and electrocoagulation) result in tumour control equivalent to that of radical surgery, but without the need for a major operation or a permanent colostomy. Survival and local recurrence appear to be similar with different forms of local therapy. Local excision has advantages because it provides a specimen to confirm the diagnosis, assess the completeness of the excision, and stage the depth of tumour penetration in the rectal wall. Results from

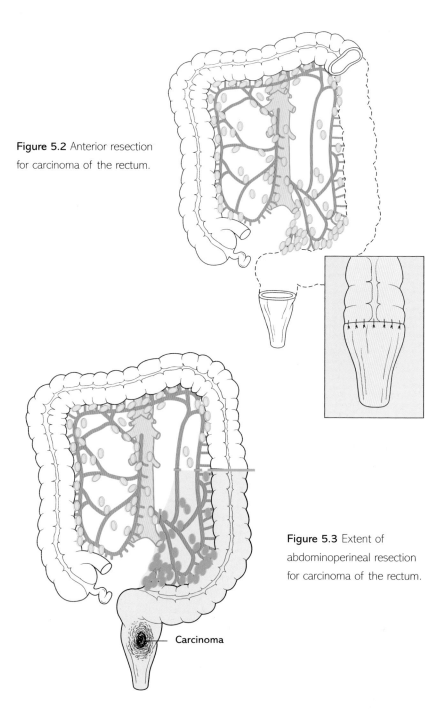

Figure 5.2 Anterior resection for carcinoma of the rectum.

Figure 5.3 Extent of abdominoperineal resection for carcinoma of the rectum.

Carcinoma

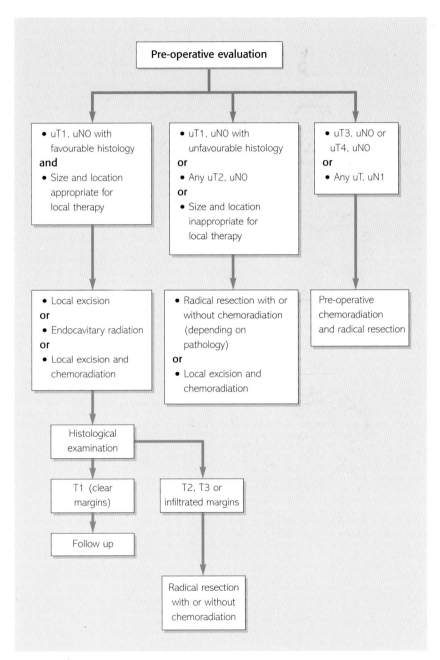

Figure 5.4 Management plan for local therapy of rectal cancer. See Table 1.2 (pages 12–13) for definitions of TNM staging acronyms.

several series following similar selection criteria report a local recurrence rate ranging from 0–26%. Half of these local recurrences can be salvaged by radical surgery. Locally advanced rectal cancers without evidence of distant metastasis should be treated aggressively with a combination of pre-operative chemoradiation therapy, radical surgery and postoperative adjuvant chemotherapy.

Mortality and morbidity. The operative mortality in patients undergoing radical surgery for rectal cancer is low, but the morbidity is significant. In addition to the complications common to any patients undergoing major abdominal procedures (atelectasis, wound infection, deep venous thrombosis) these patients are at risk for several specific complications. They include ureteral injury, pelvic haemorrhage, urinary dysfunction, impotence and retrograde ejaculation in men, dyspareunia in women, anastomotic leak in patients with low anastomosis, and perineal wound infection in patients undergoing abdominoperineal resection.

Adjuvant therapy. Up to half of the patients undergoing curative resection for rectal cancer will develop recurrent disease. The limitation of surgical resection imposed by the pelvic anatomy is responsible for local recurrence rates of up to 25% for stage II and stage III rectal cancers treated by surgery alone. In recent years, the combined administration of adjuvant radiation therapy and chemotherapy (fluorouracil), given before or after surgery, has become standard in patients with stage II and III rectal cancers. Both pre- and postoperative radiotherapy have demonstrated efficacy in local tumour control.

The rationale for the pre-operative schedule is based on the assumption that radiation therapy:
- is more effective in tumours with an intact blood supply
- can reduce cancer cell viability and the potential for dissemination at the time of surgery
- will minimize the risk of radiation enteritis in a freely mobile small bowel
- reduces tumour size and increases the probability of having a sphincter-saving procedure.

Postoperative administration of adjuvant therapy allows selection of patients at high risk of local recurrence. The new staging techniques, particularly endorectal ultrasound, now allow the pre-operative selection of patients at risk.

Several European randomized trials have shown that short-course pre-operative radiation therapy (25 Gy over 5 days) reduces local recurrence and may improve overall survival in patients who had radical surgery for rectal cancer. The effect on local control is evident even in patients who had total mesorectal excision. In the USA a dose of 50.4 Gy given over 5 weeks with concomitant administration of continuous fluorouracil infusion is the preferred treatment. The two regimens of pre-operative adjuvant therapy – short-course and long-course radiation – have never been prospectively compared. Patients with ultrasound stage II and stage III rectal cancers have a significant risk of distant recurrence and should also receive systemic adjuvant fluorouracil and leucovorin chemotherapy after recovering from surgery.

Large bowel obstruction is a common complication of colorectal cancer and requires prompt diagnosis and treatment. Obstruction develops in 7–29% of patients with colorectal cancer, and is the presenting symptom in up to 15% of patients. Large bowel obstruction is defined as mechanical blockage to the passage of colonic or rectal content with consequent abdominal distension and obstipation. Mechanical obstruction should be distinguished from acute colonic pseudo-obstruction, in which colonic and abdominal distension is caused by a functional rather than a mechanical process.

Aetiology

Colorectal cancer is responsible for 60–90% of all cases of acute colonic obstruction. Most obstructions occur in the left colon where the faeces are solid, the lumen is smaller, and the tumours are more likely to be annular. Bowel obstructions secondary to volvulus have a significant geographical variation. Volvulus is rare in the western world, but is responsible for half of all large bowel obstructions in developing countries. Large bowel obstruction secondary to diverticular disease is uncommon, and other causes are extremely rare.

The aetiology of acute colonic pseudo-obstruction is unknown, but it is frequently associated with systemic illness, trauma, prolonged immobilization, retroperitoneal pathology, constipating medications, electrolyte imbalance, endocrine disorders and colonic inflammation (Table 6.1).

Pathophysiology

The obstructed bowel undergoes significant changes in motility, secretion and blood flow, which are responsible for the clinical manifestations. Proximal to the obstructed segment, particularly in left-sided obstructions, the colon develops mass action contractions, responsible for the colic pain. Persistent obstruction and progressive distension leads to colonic hypomotility (Table 6.2).

TABLE 6.1

Aetiology of colonic obstruction and clinical conditions predisposing to colonic pseudo-obstruction

Colonic (mechanical) obstruction	Pseudo-obstruction
• Colorectal cancer	• Idiopathic (Ogilvie's syndrome)
• Diverticulitis	• Systemic illness
• Volvulus	• Pharmacological agents
• Hernia	– opioids
• Inflammatory bowel disease	– tranquillizers
	– anticholinergics
• Peritoneal neoplasias	– antidepressants
• Radiation stricture	• Immobility
• Anastomotic stricture	• Retroperitoneal pathology
• Adhesions	• Transplant recipients
• Foreign bodies	• Electrolyte imbalance
• Faecal impaction	• Colonic inflammation
	• Endocrine dysfunction

TABLE 6.2

Mechanical aspects of large bowel obstruction

- Increased motility proximal to obstruction
- Emptying of distal bowel
- Distension of proximal bowel
  - increased secretions
  - nitrogen and hydrogen sulphide gas due to bacterial overgrowth
- Bacterial translocation

Colonic obstruction causes progressive abdominal distension as a result of the accumulation of gas (mostly nitrogen from swallowed air), increased fluid secretion and hyperproliferation of anaerobic bacterial species. The accumulation of fluid in the distended colon can lead to dehydration.

Progressive distension in the presence of a competent ileocaecal valve results in a closed-loop obstruction. The increase in intraluminal pressure can compromise the mucosal blood flow and lead to irreversible ischaemia. The tension in the wall of the distended bowel increases in proportion to the fourth power of the radius and so the development of ischaemia and the risk of subsequent perforation are high, particularly in the caecum, which is the segment of the colon with the largest diameter. The risk of perforation is related not only to the calibre of the colon, but also to the onset of obstruction (higher risk when acute) and the duration of the obstruction.

Mucosal ischaemia has been implicated as the cause of a non-specific form of colitis that develops in some patients proximal to the site of obstruction. The mucosal inflammation, which can only be diagnosed at the time of surgery, should influence the extent of resection.

Diagnosis

It is sometimes difficult to distinguish acute colonic obstruction from colonic pseudo-obstruction.

Acute colonic obstruction. Patients manifest:
- abdominal discomfort or frank pain (depending on the onset of the obstruction)
- reduction or complete cessation of the passage of flatus and faeces
- progressive abdominal distension.

Auscultation of bowel sounds is rarely helpful in the diagnosis of large bowel obstruction. Abdominal tenderness, particularly if associated with fever and leukocytosis, requires immediate evaluation to exclude perforation or ischaemia. Obstructing rectal cancers are unusual and, in most patients with large bowel obstruction, digital rectal examination reveals an empty rectum.

Colonic pseudo-obstruction can cause symptoms similar to those of acute colonic obstruction. Diagnosis of colonic pseudo-obstruction can be suggested by the:
- clinical setting (immobilization, opioids, electrolyte imbalance)
- passage of small amounts of gas and faeces
- lack of tenderness in a massively distended abdomen.

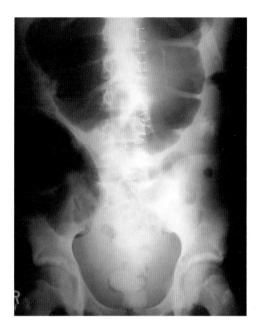

Figure 6.1 Radiograph showing colonic distension.

However, the definitive diagnosis often requires specific radiological tests, such as a water-soluble contrast enema.

Diagnostic tests

A number of tests are used to aid diagnosis, including:

- radiography
- water-soluble contrast enema
- colonoscopy
- endoscopy
- abdominal CT.

The plain abdominal film demonstrates colonic distension, with air fluid levels, and a cut-off at the site of obstruction (Figure 6.1). The absence of small bowel distension indicates a competent ileocaecal valve, with the increased risk of caecal perforation. The presence of gas in the small bowel and rectum raises the possibility of ileus or colonic pseudo-obstruction, but the radiological findings can be misleading (Figure 6.2). The presence of intramural gas indicates advanced ischaemia. A chest radiograph should always be obtained to exclude the presence of pneumoperitoneum.

Figure 6.2 Radiograph showing gas in the small bowel.

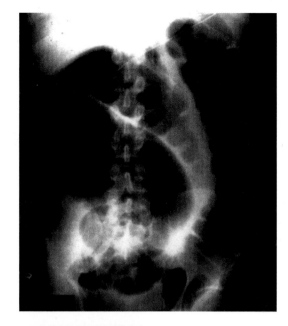

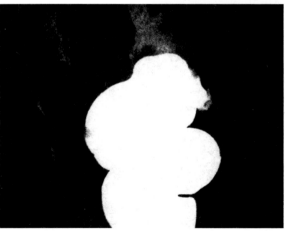

Figure 6.3 Gastrographin enema demonstrating obstruction of the rectosigmoid junction.

Water-soluble contrast enema. This test helps to determine the degree and level of obstruction (Figure 6.3). The flow of contrast to the caecum and the absence of mucosal abnormalities suggests colonic pseudo-obstruction. The osmotic effect of the water-soluble contrast material may have a therapeutic effect in decompressing the colon in these patients. The mucosal detail at the site of obstruction may help to define the cause of the obstruction.

Colonoscopy is a better alternative to contrast enema when confirming the presence of cancer. It may be therapeutic in cases of obstruction secondary to volvulus.

Abdominal CT may be useful to exclude diverticulitis as the potential cause of obstruction. A CT pneumocolon can demonstrate the site and cause of obstruction as well as provide information about the extent of malignant spread.

Treatment

Patients presenting with obstructing colorectal cancer have a higher operative mortality and morbidity, and a poorer long-term prognosis than patients undergoing elective resection. Therefore, the goal of surgery is to reduce mortality and morbidity and obtain functional results similar to those obtained in patients undergoing elective resection.

In the absence of perforation, the main differences between patients with obstructing and non-obstructing lesions are:
- the pathophysiological consequences of obstruction (dehydration, respiratory compromise, ischaemic colitis)
- the inability to prepare the proximal colon
- the technical difficulties imposed by a massively distended bowel.

The surgical approach should aim to correct these factors.

Pre-operative fluid resuscitation and correction of electrolyte imbalances are important in patients with large bowel obstruction. A urinary catheter facilitates fluid management. Unstable patients should be appropriately monitored in the intensive care unit. A nasogastric tube prevents accumulation of swallowed air. Antibiotic prophylaxis with a second-generation cephalosporin or a combination of an aminoglycoside and metronidazole should be given at the time of surgery. Peri-operative morbidity and mortality are three times higher with surgery performed for obstruction compared with elective surgery. Cardiopulmonary complications and abdominal sepsis are the major causes of in-hospital mortality and morbidity.

Surgical management depends on the location of the obstruction. Lesions proximal to the splenic flexure are commonly treated by an extended right hemicolectomy with primary anastomosis between the terminal ileum and the non-obstructed colon distal to the lesion. This has the advantage of being a single procedure, removing the entire segment of distended and potentially ischaemic bowel, and eliminating the risk of leaving a synchronous tumour in the obstructed colon. Some of these patients develop mild, but usually temporary, diarrhoea.

The management of a lesion located distal to the splenic flexure is more controversial (Table 6.3). The three-stage approach is rarely performed today. Resection of the segment containing the tumour, closure of the rectal stump as a Hartmann's pouch, and construction of an end colostomy, followed by bowel anastomosis at a later date, has been a popular choice in the last decades. However, the cumulative mortality and morbidity of both

TABLE 6.3

Surgical alternatives in the treatment of malignant left colon obstruction

Emergency surgery
Three-stage procedure
- Diverting colostomy
- Resection and anastomosis
- Closure of colostomy

Two-stage procedure
- Primary resection, end-colostomy and Hartmann's pouch
- Colorectal anastomosis

One-stage procedures
- Subtotal colectomy and ileorectal anastomosis

or

- Segmental colectomy, intraoperative colon lavage, primary anastomosis

Non-surgical decompression and elective surgery
- YAG laser

or

- Intraluminal stent

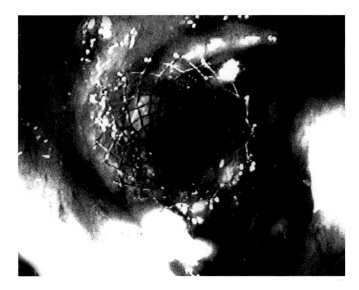

Figure 6.4
Expandable
endoluminal
prosthesis.

procedures is significant, and at least 30% of patients are left with a
permanent colostomy. This operation is now limited to situations in which
a primary anastomosis is contraindicated (e.g. in the presence of faecal
peritonitis from an obstructed and perforated tumour).

The goal today is to relieve the obstruction and treat the cancer in a
single operative procedure. Options include:

- treating the obstruction pre-operatively, and then preparing the colon for
  an elective procedure
- subtotal colectomy and ileorectal anastomosis
- segmental resection, on-table lavage of the obstructed segment and
  primary anastomosis.

Non-operative colonic decompression. The obstruction can be relieved
pre-operatively by either endoluminal resection of the tumour with the help
of a YAG laser, or by placement of an expandable endoluminal prosthesis
(Figure 6.4). Both procedures relieve the obstruction, and allow non-
operative decompression and mechanical preparation of the colon. This
enables elective resection to take place during the same admission. Although
no comparative studies have been performed between these techniques, the
placement of an endoluminal prosthesis is technically simple and available
in most hospitals. These techniques are contraindicated when there are signs
of perforation or colonic ischaemia.

Subtotal colectomy with ileorectal anastomosis is a quick operation, reduces the risk of leaving behind a synchronous tumour in the obstructed portion of the colon, minimizes the risk of faecal spillage, uses non-distended bowel for the anastomosis and facilitates the follow-up of these patients. The disadvantages, however, are a higher incidence of bowel obstruction after ileorectal anastomosis and the development of diarrhoea that may become incapacitating in elderly patients.

Segmental resection with intraoperative colonic lavage and primary anastomosis is a smaller operation and avoids the risk of diarrhoea. Disadvantages are the risk of faecal spillage, the use of distended colon for the anastomosis, and the possibility of leaving a synchronous tumour in the obstructed segment of the colon.

Although surgical tradition has condemned the performance of an anastomosis in an unprepared colon, experience accumulated from the management of patients with civilian colon trauma has demonstrated that, under specific circumstances, a primary anastomosis can be performed safely in unprepared colon. This experience has been transferred to malignant colonic obstruction.

Approximately 50% of patients with colorectal cancer present with advanced disease unsuitable for curative surgery. Nevertheless, the majority of these patients will have resectable tumours for which surgery is clearly indicated. Surgery is performed frequently as a palliative measure to prevent symptoms of obstruction or bleeding, or to relieve these symptoms. Even tumours that are densely adherent to adjacent structures (e.g. the abdominal wall, bladder or small bowel) should be considered for resectional surgery. Studies of the resection of large tumours have demonstrated significant benefits in terms of palliation and enhancement of symptom-free survival.

Recurrence

Approximately half of the patients who have undergone surgery for colorectal cancer will develop a recurrence, the majority within 3 years of initial resection. The management of these patients should be decided in a multidisciplinary setting of surgeons, medical oncologists, radiotherapists, radiologists and pathologists. Such multidisciplinary groups are becoming increasingly popular and have demonstrated their value.

The pattern of recurrence for colorectal cancer is fairly standard. Patients present with:

- liver metastases
- local recurrence
- a combination of local recurrence and liver metastases
- peritoneal recurrence
- lung metastases
- widespread distant metastases (although this is rare).

Liver metastases

Approximately 25% of patients with colorectal cancer have liver metastases present at the time of initial presentation. Of the remainder, 50% will develop a recurrence with the liver as the major site of metastases (Figure 7.1).

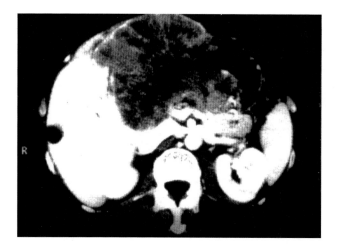

Figure 7.1 CT scan of liver showing extensive metastasis involving the left and part of the right lobe of the liver.

Investigation of patients with colorectal liver metastases should determine whether the metastatic disease is resectable. Approximately 10% of patients with colorectal liver metastases have disease confined to a single lobe. Even if there are several metastases in one lobe, surgery should be considered. Surgery for resection may involve either a segmentectomy or hemi-hepatectomy (Figure 7.2). These procedures can be carried out with an operative mortality of less than 5%. Recent studies have shown that 3-year survival following resection is approximately 60% and 5-year survival approximately 25%. It is important to ensure that patients have disease confined to the liver prior to consideration of resection (Table 7.1).

In patients with multiple liver metastases unsuitable for resection, the following therapeutic modalities must be considered.

TABLE 7.1

Selection criteria for resection of liver metastases

- Preferably confined to single lobe
- No extrahepatic metastases
- Patient fit for major surgery
- Non-jaundiced
- Good liver function
- No local recurrence

Systemic chemotherapy. An effective and widely used chemotherapy regimen is the combination of fluorouracil and leucovorin, given as an infusion. The response rate for this regimen is approximately 20%, and there is evidence of an improvement in survival. Systemic chemotherapy improves palliation in this group of patients and can be delivered with few toxic side-effects. Systemic chemotherapy is delivered at 2-week intervals. New cytotoxic agents are being developed, and others are being assessed in randomized clinical trials. Raltitrexed (Tomudex®) directly inhibits thymidylate synthase. It can be administered by an intravenous bolus every

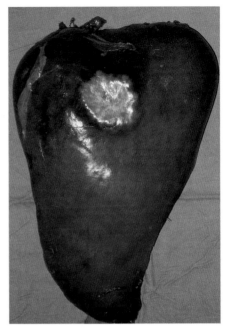

Figure 7.2 Resection specimen following right hemi-hepatectomy for localized liver metastasis.

3 weeks, and has been compared with bolus fluorouracil and leucovorin. Tumour response rates appear to be similar.

Two other drugs deserve comment. Irinotecan, a DNA topoisomerase I inhibitor, has been used for years as a second-line agent and recently as a first line of therapy in patients with advanced colorectal cancer. Irinotecan has been used as a second-line therapy in patients with metastatic disease not responding to fluorouracil and calcium leucovorin (calcium folinate). The response rate in this setting was 20% to 30%, with a median duration of response of 6.7 months. In the first-line setting, two prospective randomized trials have shown that irinotecan combined with fluorouracil and calcium leucovorin increases the response rate and the median survival in patients with metastatic colorectal cancer compared with fluorouracil and calcium leucovorin alone. Consequently, irinotecan combined with fluorouracil and calcium leucovorin is now considered the new standard therapy for patients with metastatic colorectal cancer.

Oxaliplatin induces apoptotic cell death, and is active in the presence of infusional fluorouracil and leucovorin. Randomized trials have shown improved response and progression-free survival when added to fluorouracil and leucovorin. There is evidence that oxaliplatin is beneficial in down-staging extensive liver metastases and thus may allow resectional surgery to be performed resulting in improved survival.

There is no doubt that, in the near future, other drugs will be developed for advanced colorectal cancer that may subsequently have a place in the adjuvant setting.

Locoregional chemotherapy. Liver metastases obtain the majority of their blood supply from the hepatic artery. In the past 20 years, numerous studies have used locoregional hepatic arterial chemotherapy to deliver higher and more effective doses of chemotherapy directly to liver metastases. This procedure involves insertion of an arterial catheter into the hepatic artery via the gastroduodenal artery (Figure 7.3). High-dose, infusional fluorouracil and fluorourodeoxyuridine (FUDR) can be administered in this way.

Meta-analysis of studies using locoregional chemotherapy has demonstrated an overall improvement in survival compared with systemic chemotherapy. However in a recent trial, a combination of intrahepatic arterial fluorouracil chemotherapy and systemic leucovorin compared with systemic chemotherapy was unable to demonstrate a significant benefit in overall survival. Since there is morbidity associated with the insertion of implantable intrahepatic devices, this technique cannot be recommended as

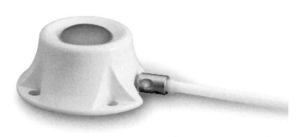

Figure 7.3 A Port-a-Cath® for insertion into the hepatic artery to deliver locoregional chemotherapy to the liver. Photograph courtesy of Deltec, Inc., St Paul, MN, USA.

a routine outside clinical trials. The more recently developed systemic drugs appear to be more effective than previous regimens in the treatment of metastatic disease.

Interstitial treatment. It is possible to destroy liver tumours *in situ* in selected patients by:

- cryotherapy
- interstitial laser photocoagulation
- radiofrequency ablation
- local injection of alcohol.

Each of these techniques has its advocates. There have been reports of improvement in survival following selective interstitial therapy, but it is important to select patients carefully and to realize that present evidence shows these techniques to be purely palliative. Nevertheless, there is increasing enthusiasm for radiofrequency ablation of liver metastases combined with systemic chemotherapy or in association with a policy of liver resection. Major liver metastases can be resected and smaller geographically distant ones in the liver can be dealt with by radiofrequency destruction.

Treatment of locally recurrent colon and rectal cancer

Pelvic recurrence is a devastating problem in patients who have undergone 'curative' resection for rectal cancer. Local recurrence is a cause of major disability. It carries a very poor prognosis and has a median survival of only 13 months. Uncontrolled pelvic recurrence can be the source of significant pain, tenesmus and distress from the presence and smell of a necrotic tumour protruding through the perineum.

The reported incidence of isolated local recurrence is 3–32%. This variation between series is due not only to factors that affect the risk of local recurrence, but also to differences in the length of follow-up and diagnostic criteria.

Recurrent rectal cancer treatment results are poor, and therefore prevention is one of the main forms of treatment. Prevention may be achieved by choosing the appropriate operation for the stage of the tumour, by using meticulous surgical technique, and by the use of adequate adjuvant therapy. Surgical technique is a significant factor and with increasing appreciation of total mesorectal excision the incidence of recurrent disease should fall.

Surgery. Autopsy series report that 25–50% of patients with local recurrence have cancer confined to the pelvis when they die, and therefore an aggressive treatment in these patients seems justified.

The extent of surgery depends on:

- the primary operation
- prior use of adjuvant therapy
- the size and location of the recurrence.

Surgery often involves resection of adjacent pelvic organs such as the uterus, vagina, bladder, ureter and sacrum, and bony structures of the pelvic wall. These operations usually require extensive reconstructive surgery. Contraindications for resective surgery include the presence of distant metastases, extensive involvement of the pelvic wall, iliac–venous obstruction and bilateral sciatic pain.

Less than half of those patients who have exploratory laparotomy for local recurrence undergo curative resection. Less than one-third of patients undergoing resection survive 5 years.

Intraoperative radiation therapy combined with aggressive surgery may improve tumour control and increase survival in patients undergoing palliative or curative surgical resection for locally recurrent rectal cancer.

Occasionally, recurrence can result in fistulas to the bladder (colovesical fistulas), vagina (colovaginal fistulas) or the abdominal wall. These are serious problems and patients may require palliative surgery, such as colostomy.

An aggressive surgical approach is also warranted for those few patients who develop an isolated local recurrence after surgical treatment of colon cancer. Long-term survival or sustained palliation can be achieved with surgical resection of local recurrences not involving vital structures.

Multimodal therapy. Some groups have developed a combined protocol to treat previously non-irradiated, biopsy-proven, recurrent rectal cancer. This is based on the improved rates of resectability and the decreased incidence of local recurrence after pre-operative chemoradiation therapy for locally advanced rectal cancer. The protocol includes pre-operative chemoradiation, aggressive surgical resection, and selective intraoperative radiation. Resectability is increased and local control improved.

Radiation therapy has been the most important therapeutic modality in the management of symptomatic, non-resectable recurrent disease. Some series report up to 90% initial pain control and improved quality of life, but no impact on median survival. The addition of chemotherapy increases toxicity without improving local control.

Other palliative procedures such as stents for ureteral obstructions, colostomy in patients with rectal obstruction for pelvic recurrence, and nerve block, may offer significant palliation in selected patients.

Peritoneal metastases

It is not uncommon for patients to develop malignant ascites as a result of multiple peritoneal metastases following surgery for colorectal cancer. This form of recurrence is fatal and there are very few significant treatments to assist. Paracentesis is indicated if ascites is major and causing distressing symptoms. This may need to be repeated and is often associated with intraperitoneal instillation of chemotherapeutic agents.

Other distant metastases

It is unusual for patients with colorectal cancer to develop metastases outside the peritoneal cavity. When they do occur, the most common sites are the lung, brain and bone. These occurrences are unusual compared with liver metastases, and patients rarely develop metastases in these sites without the presence of existing liver metastases. It appears that metastases spread from metastases.

For years, surgery has been the mainstay of treatment for colorectal cancer patients. Once the diagnosis was made, the surgeon was the main, and often the only, health specialist responsible for their care. But recent advances in molecular biology, epidemiology, surgical technique, radiation therapy, chemotherapy, interventional radiology, and patient support services have resulted in new treatment options and improved clinical outcomes. Nowadays, the treatment of colorectal cancer patients often requires coordinated decision-making by several specialists from different disciplines. The need for a multidisciplinary approach to colorectal cancer is particularly evident in some specific clinical scenarios highlighted below.

Hereditary risk assessment

The discovery in the past decade of the genetic mutations responsible for the hereditary colorectal cancer syndromes, i.e. familial adenomatous polyposis (FAP) and hereditary non-polyposis colorectal cancer (HNPCC), has raised the possibility of integrating genetic testing into clinical practice. Many professional societies have now developed guidelines to help clinicians provide genetic counselling and genetic testing for patients who may have a hereditary colorectal cancer syndrome. The results of such counselling and testing would then be used as the basis for recommendations regarding not only the treatment and surveillance of the index patients, but also screening and counselling of their extended family. The extent of a colectomy in an HNPCC patient with colorectal cancer, the selection between a prophylactic colectomy or colonoscopy surveillance in an asymptomatic patient with a germline mutation in one of the MMR genes, or the timing for a colectomy in a patient with attenuated FAP, are questions that should be addressed by a multidisciplinary team, including the primary-care physician, genetic counsellor, gastroenterologist and colorectal surgeon.

The hereditary predisposition to colorectal cancer, although not as evident as in patients with FAP and HNPCC, is also important in the 25%

of patients with a family history of colorectal cancer who do not meet the diagnostic criteria for FAP or HNPCC. Close collaboration between the primary-care physician, gastroenterologist and colorectal surgeon is often required to ensure proper surveillance and appropriate screening recommendations for such patients and their families.

Treatment of primary disease

Several prospective randomized studies conducted over the past twenty years have demonstrated that fluorouracil and leucovorin given after curative-intent surgery for stage III colon cancer increase survival as compared with surgery alone. New chemotherapy agents that have proven effective for advanced disease are now being tested in the adjuvant setting. Consequently, the care of these patients requires close collaboration between the colorectal surgeon and medical oncologist.

The care of rectal cancer patients is based on pre-operative tumour staging and histological results. In recent years, stage I rectal cancer patients have been treated with local excision with (T2N0) or without (T1N0) postoperative chemoradiation. For patients with stage II or stage III rectal cancer, chemoradiation before or after surgery reduces the rate of local recurrence and possibly improves survival as compared with surgery alone. Thus the radiation oncologist has become a crucial team member.

The need for a multidisciplinary approach is particularly evident in patients who present with stage IV disease. Their treatment must be planned individually, taking into consideration the disease-related symptoms, the overall patient medical condition, the potential consequences of progression of the primary lesion, and the extent and resectability of the metastatic disease. The selection and the timing of the different treatment options – whether surgery, chemotherapy, radiation therapy, or any combination of them – must involve the colorectal surgeon, medical oncologist, radiation oncologist, hepatobiliary surgeon and thoracic surgeon.

Recurrent disease

Metastatic disease can rarely be addressed by a single specialist. A hepatobiliary surgeon may resect an isolated liver metastasis, or a thoracic surgeon a lung metastasis, but most patients with metastatic disease are usually candidates for several forms of therapy involving more than one specialty. For example, a patient with multiple liver metastases may need systemic chemotherapy, hepatic artery infusional chemotherapy, radiofrequency ablation, or even surgery.

Fortunately, isolated pelvic recurrences after curative-intent surgery for rectal cancer are infrequent. The role of radical surgery, even in patients with potentially resectable recurrent tumours, remains controversial. However, whether treated with curative-intent surgery or palliative methods, patients with pelvic recurrences require a multidisciplinary approach. In addition to surgery, most of them will need pre-operative and/or intra-operative radiation and systemic chemotherapy. Curative-intent surgery often demands a pelvic exenteration with sacrectomy; the surgical team will include not only a colorectal surgeon, but also a urologist, a neurosurgeon and a plastic surgeon. Patients treated for palliation often develop bowel or ureteral obstruction that may require input from an interventional radiologist for placement of stents or nephrostomy catheters. In patients with advanced disease the contribution of a pain specialist is of inestimable value.

A significant proportion of colorectal cancer patients may need a temporary or permanent stoma. In these patients the contribution of the stomatherapist spans aspects from the selection of the stoma site to the management of stoma complications.

The global effects of the disease and its treatment result in physical distress, physiological stress, financial burden and overall impairment in quality of life that demand the input of a sophisticated patient support system.

Conclusion

The treatment of colorectal cancer is best approached by a core multidisciplinary team integrated by the primary-care physician, colorectal surgeon, medical oncologist and radiation oncologist. The variety of clinical situations that may present in these patients often requires the contribution of an expanded team of healthcare providers from different specialties (Figure 8.1).

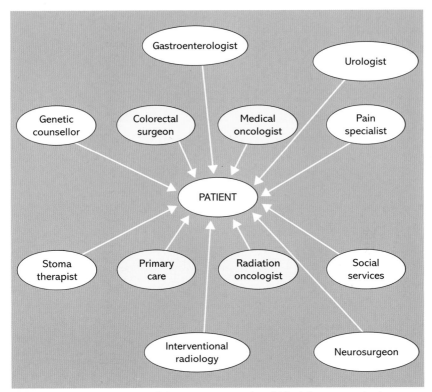

Figure 8.1 A representation of the patient-centred multidisciplinary team in the management of colorectal cancer.

Progress made in the understanding of the biology, natural history, prevention and treatment of colorectal cancer during the past decade has been rewarded with a persistent decline in the mortality from this disease. The future prospects for different areas related to this disease will probably help to accelerate this trend in coming years.

Biology. In the past decade, we have witnessed an explosion of knowledge regarding the molecular alterations responsible for the development and progression of colorectal cancer. Several oncogenes and tumour suppressor genes have been found to be mutated in colorectal cancer, and it is expected that new mutations will soon be discovered.

Attempts to correlate molecular alterations with clinical behaviour in colorectal cancers have been, for the most part, unsuccessful. The development of new genome screening tools, such as the serial analyses of gene expression and cDNA microassays, will facilitate the correlation between molecular alterations and the biological behaviour of individual colorectal cancers. This information may have prognostic value and could be used to select therapy.

Prevention. The genetic basis to the familial predisposition has become more evident in recent years, but there is a large body of evidence supporting the influence of several environmental factors in the development of colorectal cancer. Changes in some of these factors, such as decreasing fat and increasing fibre intakes, and the use of calcium and vitamin C supplements, may reduce the incidence of colorectal cancer. There is increasing evidence of a protective effect of non-steroidal anti-inflammatory drugs (NSAIDs). Gene-knockout studies in mice suggest that inhibition of the cyclooxygenase type 2 pathway by NSAIDs may be important.

Screening. Although the FOB test has low sensitivity, poor specificity and poor predictive value, its use as a screening tool has been shown to reduce the mortality from colorectal cancer. Screening with flexible sigmoidoscopy is likely to have the same effect. However, the impact of screening on the incidence of colorectal cancer has been minimal, as the percentage of screened adults remains very low. Screening is expensive, and the implementation of the present guidelines may be logistically and financially impracticable. Therefore we need to identify groups at risk that will make screening cost effective. In the future, improved screening tools will replace the FOB test.

Diagnosis. The combination of spiral CT and virtual-reality computer technology has resulted in a new method of colonic examination called 'virtual colonoscopy'. This may have a significant impact on the acceptance and safety of colorectal cancer screening and diagnosis. Other diagnostic modalities, such as positron emission tomography (PET) scanning and MRI will have a role in the diagnosis and staging of colorectal cancer.

Treatment. Laparoscopic colon resection for cancer has been proved to be technically feasible and functionally and cosmetically advantageous for the patient. Whether it is oncologically equivalent to open resection will be determined by several prospective studies now in course.

Radical resection with an adequate distal margin combined with pre-operative or postoperative chemoradiation is the standard treatment of locally advanced rectal cancer. However, the universal adoption of the technique of total mesorectal excision may make radiation unnecessary, at least in patients with T3 rectal tumours.

Adjuvant therapy for colorectal cancer is based on fluorouracil combined with levamisole, leucovorin or radiation. Several new drugs, such as the thymidylate synthase inhibitors, the topoisomerase I inhibitors, ethynyluracil, oxaliplatin and fluorouracil prodrugs, some of which are already in phase III trials, may change this spectrum in the near future. Other promising therapeutic alternatives include angiogenesis inhibitors, matrix-metalloproteinase inhibitors, apoptosis-promoting drugs and specific immunotherapy.

There is also increasing interest in gene therapy designed to correct mutations which effect the growth of tumour cells. In one study, adenovirus encoding wild-type *p53* has been delivered by hepatic artery infusion to patients with *p53*-mutated colorectal liver metastases.

Key references

DIAGNOSIS AND STAGING

Deen KI, Madoff RD, Belmonte C et al. Preoperative staging of rectal neoplasms with endorectal ultrasonography. *Sem Colon Rectal Surg* 1995;6:78–85.

Mulcahey HE, O'Donoghue DP. Duration of colorectal cancer symptoms and survival: the effect of confounding clinical and pathological variables. *Eur J Cancer* 1997;33:1461–7.

Rex DK, Rahmani EY, Haseman JH et al. Relative sensitivity of colonoscopy and barium enema for detection of colorectal cancer in clinical practice. *Gastroenterology* 1997;112:17–23.

Royster AP, Fenlon HM, Clarke PD et al. CT colonoscopy of colorectal neoplasms: two-dimensional virtual-reality techniques with colonoscopic correlation. *Am J Roentgenol* 1997;169:1237–42.

Schnall MD, Furth EE, Rosato EE et al. Rectal tumor stage: correlation of endorectal MR imaging and pathologic findings. Comment in: *Radiology* 1994;190:663–5.

Zerhouni EA, Rutter C, Hamilton SR et al. CT and MR imaging in the staging of colorectal carcinoma: report of the Radiology Diagnostic Oncology Group II. *Radiology* 1996;200:443–51.

SCREENING AND HIGH-RISK PATIENTS

Ahlquist DA, Skoletsky JE, Boynton KA et al. Colorectal cancer screening by detection of altered human DNA in stool: feasibility of a multitarget assay panel. *Gastroenterology* 2000;119:1219–27.

Fuchs CS, Giovannucci EL, Colditz GA et al. A prospective study of family history and the risk of colorectal cancer. *N Engl J Med* 1994;331:1669–74.

Hardcastle JD, Chamberlain J, Sheffield J et al. Randomised, controlled trial of faecal occult blood screening for colorectal cancer. Results for first 107,349 subjects. *Lancet* 1989;1:1160–4.

Kewenter J, Björk S, Haglind E et al. Screening and rescreening of colorectal cancer: a controlled trial of fecal occult blood testing in 27,700 subjects. *Cancer* 1988;62:645–751.

Kronborg O, Fenger C, Olsen J et al. Repeated screening for colorectal cancer with fecal occult blood test: a prospective randomized study at Funen, Denmark. *Scand J Gastroenterol* 1989;24:599–606.

Lieberman DA, Weiss DG, Bond JH et al. Use of colonoscopy to screen asymptomatic adults for colorectal cancer. *N Engl J Med* 2000;343:162–8.

Mandel JS, Bond JH, Church TR et al. Reducing mortality from colorectal cancer by screening for fecal occult blood. *N Engl J Med* 1993;328:1365–71.

Selby JV, Friedman GD, Quesenberry CP et al. A case-control study of screening sigmoidoscopy and mortality from colorectal cancer. N Engl J Med 1992; 326:653–7.

Winawer SJ, Fletcher RH, Miller L et al. Colorectal cancer screening: clinical guidelines and rationale. Gastroenterology 1997;112:594–642.

Winawer SJ, Zauber AG, Ho MN et al. Prevention of colorectal cancer by colonoscopic polypectomy. N Engl J Med 1993;329:1977–81.

Winawer SJ, Zauber AG, O'Brien MJ et al. Randomized comparison of surveillance intervals after colonoscopic removal of newly diagnosed adenomatous polyps. N Engl J Med 1993;328:901–6.

TREATMENT OF PRIMARY DISEASE

Chung-Faye GA, Kerr DJ. Innovative treatment for colon cancer. BMJ 2000;321:1397–9.

Eckhauser FE, Knol JA. Surgery for primary and metastatic colorectal cancer (Review). Gastroenterol Clin North Am 1997;26:103–28.

Enker WE, Havenga K, Polyak T et al. Abdominoperineal resection via total mesorectal excision and autonomic nerve presentation for low rectal cancer. World J Surg 1997;21:715–20.

Fazio VW, Tjandra JJ. Primary therapy of carcinoma of the large bowel. World J Surg 1991;15:568–75.

Kapiteijn E, Marijnen CAM, Nagtegaal ID et al. Preoperative radiotherapy combined with total mesorectal excision for resectable rectal cancer. N Engl J Med 2001;345:638–46.

Langman M, Boyle P. Chemoprevention of colorectal cancer. Gut 1998;43:578–85.

Lavery JC, Lopez-Kostner F, Fazio VW et al. Chances of cure are not compromised with sphincter-saving procedures for cancer of the lower third of the rectum. Surgery 1997;122:779–85.

MacFarlane JK, Ryall RDH, Heald RJ. Mesorectal excision for rectal cancer. Lancet 1993;341:457–60.

NIH Consensus Conference. Adjuvant therapy for patients with colon and rectal cancer. JAMA 1990;246:1444–50.

Roth JA, Cristiano RJ. Cancer: what have we done and where are we going? J Natl Cancer Inst 1997;89:21–39.

Swedish Rectal Cancer Trial. Improved survival with preoperative radiotherapy in resectable rectal cancer. N Engl J Med 1997;336:980–7.

The International Multicentre Pooled Analysis of B2 Colon Cancer Trials (IMPACT B2) Investigators. Efficacy of adjuvant fluorouracil and folinic acid in B2 colon cancer. J Clin Oncol 1999;17:1356–63.

LARGE BOWEL OBSTRUCTION

Baron TH, Dean PA, Yates MR et al. Expandable metal stents for the treatment of colonic obstruction: techniques and outcomes. Gastrointest Endosc 1998; 47:277–86.

Deans GT, Krukowski ZH, Irwin T. Malignant obstruction of the left colon. Br J Surg 1994;81:1270–6.

Eckhauser ML. Laser therapy of colorectal carcinoma. Surg Clin North Am 1992; 72:597–607.

Rex DK. Colonoscopy and acute colonic pseudo-obstruction. *Gastrointest Endosc Clin North Am* 1997;7:499–507.

The Scotia Study Group. Single-stage treatment for malignant left-sided colonic obstruction: a prospective randomized clinical trial comparing subtotal colectomy with segmental resection following intraoperative irrigation. *Br J Surg* 1995;82:1622–7.

ADVANCED AND RECURRENT DISEASE

Cunningham D, Findlay M. The chemotherapy of colon cancer can no longer be ignored. *Eur J Cancer* 1996;29A:2077–9.

Cunningham D, Pyrhonen S, James RD *et al.* Randomised trial of irinotecan plus supportive care versus supportive care alone after fluorouracil failure for patients with metastatic colorectal cancer. *Lancet* 1998;352:1413–18.

De Gramont A, Figer A, Seymour M *et al.* Leucovorin and fluorouracil with or without oxaliplatin as first-line treatment in advanced colorectal cancer. *J Clin Oncol* 2000;18:2938–47.

Douillard JY, Cunningham D *et al.* Irinotecan combined with fluorouracil compared with fluorouracil alone as first-line treatment for metastatic colorectal cancer – a multicentre randomised trial. *Lancet* 2000;355:1041–7.

Piedbois P. Adjuvant treatment of colon cancer. *Semin Oncol* 2000;28(suppl):1–49.

Scheithauer W, Rosen H, Kornek GV *et al.* Randomised comparison of combination chemotherapy plus supportive care or supportive care alone in patients with metastatic colorectal cancer. *BMJ* 1993;306:752–5.

The Advanced Colorectal Cancer Meta-analysis Project. Modulation of fluorouracil by leucovorin in patients with advanced colorectal cancer: evidence in terms of response rate. *J Clin Oncol* 1992;10: 896–903.

The Nordic Gastrointestinal Tumor Adjuvant Project. Expectancy or primary chemotherapy in patients with advanced asymptomatic colorectal cancer: a randomised trial. *J Clin Oncol* 1992; 10:904–11.

MULTIDISCIPLINARY MANAGEMENT

Minsky BD. Multidisciplinary case teams: an approach to the future management of advanced colororetal cancer. *Br J Cancer* 1988;77(suppl 2):1–4.

Rougier P, Neoptolemos JP. The need for a multidisciplinary approach in the treatment of advanced colorectal cancer: a critical review from a medical oncologist and surgeon. *Eur J Surg Oncol* 1997;23: 385–96.

Useful websites

The following is a list of some useful websites published by patient-support, research-funding or healthcare professional organizations.

American Society of Colon and Rectal Surgeons
www.fascrs.org

Beating Bowel Cancer
www.bowelcancer.org

British Colostomy Association
www.bcass.org.uk

CancerBACUP
www.bacup.org.uk

Cancerlinks: Colorectal Cancer
www.cancerlinks.com/colorectal.html

CancerNet™
www.cancernet.nci.nih.gov

Cancer Research UK
(uniting the Cancer Research Campaign and the Imperial Cancer Research Fund)
www.cancerresearchuk.org

Hereditary Bowel Cancer
www.mdanderson.org/depts/hcc

Ileostomy and Internal Pouch Support Group
www.ileostomypouch.demon.co.uk

National Association for Colitis and Crohn's Disease
www.nacc.org.uk

National Cancer Institute
www.nci.nih.gov

Index